Eat Like A Hero

Save Lives With Your Fork

Andrea Laurel

Dear Qyenetta,
Thank you for
sharing your
light!
Best,
Andrea

This book is dedicated to the City of Plantation Fire Department in Plantation, Florida.

Without you, I wouldn't have given so much thought to saving lives and preserving property.

Because of you, I have put my time and my heart into exactly that.

Thank you.

Acknowledgements:

Much gratitude goes to my editor and mother Josie Sanfeliu, President of Latinas Against FDNY Cuts. She did a tremendous and meticulous job. Her computer and language skills were much appreciated. Such a project required great attention to detail. She spent countless patient hours on this book, and did a great job. No solid achievement is done entirely alone, and I thank God for that!

Appreciation also goes out to my significant other, fiancé, dietary test subject, proofreader, and Driver/Engineer/Inspector Eric Steinberg. His ongoing support is paramount. His critical eye helped to make this a better read for you. It was his idea to offer you greater inspiration and support via the website. Thank you, Tech Support!

Disclaimer:

This book contains suggestions and references based on the author's personal observations, research and experience. Please take personal responsibility for your own health. The author and publisher assume no liability for your actions. Please consult with your own healthcare professional to determine the best course of action for treating and preventing disease.

TABLE OF CONTENTS

"All truth passes through three stages. First, it is ridiculed. Second, it is violently opposed. Third, it is accepted as being self-evident." –Arthur Schopenhauer, German Philosopher (1788-1860)

INTRODUCTION

There are plenty of excellent reasons for anyone to switch to a plant based diet. Better health and disease prevention are great personal and family reasons. Sparing factory farmed animals' misery is altruistic. Using our earth's resources sustainably works for our society now and for future generations. Avoiding meat with bird flu, salmonella, mad cow, parasites, hormones, antibiotics and radiation is good common sense. Awareness of agribusiness lobbying and subsidies affects you not just as a taxpayer, but as a consumer. Using crops to fatten livestock while humans are starving to death is a lesson in misplaced priorities. Knowledge of our place in the community as role models and heroes should help spur us on to do the right thing. Your taste buds will adjust to a higher authority. Many champion athletes, world leaders and visionaries have plant based diets. Our daily dietary decisions have rippling

1

consequences that affect your crew, our community, our nation and our planet. You can save lives and preserve property with your fork.

BUT HUMANS ARE NATURALLY MEAT EATERS...I NEED MY PROTEIN... AND OTHER MYTHS

Well, if that were true, then we would have only canine teeth, claws and short digestive systems. If we were meant to eat meat, we would have many sharp teeth to tear and rip flesh, like a dog or a bear. We would eat our animals alive and raw. Our intestines would be short like a carnivore. Instead, we have teeth more similar to herbivores and omnivores, and a very long digestive system. For more on comparative anatomy of herbivores and carnivores, see: VegSource.[1] Much of the animal meat that we eat such as beef is 'aged' or rotted. Mold caps grow over the meat and the mold's bacteria breaks down and tenderizes the meat with enzymes. In nature, meat that is aged or rotted is eaten by vultures, hyenas and maggots. Our primate relatives eat mostly greens and fruits. Monkeys, chimpanzees, orangutans, and gorillas eat occasional bugs, but primarily survive on fruit and vegetables. In nature, animals eat food right off the tree or from the ground. True carnivores eat their prey fresh and raw. Here's

3

a test: If you give a toddler an apple and a bunny, and he eats the bunny, you've got a natural carnivore.

Protein is readily available in vegetables. There is more bioavailable protein in broccoli, kale or spinach than in steak, chicken or fish. Protein is also found in nuts, seeds and legumes. We can obtain protein by eating animals that eat greens, but then we also ingest the animal's fat which deposits and congeals on our artery walls, forming plaque. People eat protein to be 'strong as an ox', forgetting that the ox eats grass. We can just skip the animal meat and then skip the cholesterol lowering drugs too. Eating fruits and vegetables directly is more cost and resource efficient. Most Americans don't need to be concerned with getting enough protein, as on the average, we eat more twice the amount of protein recommended.[2]

"In fact, if one person is unkind to an animal it is considered to be cruelty, but where a lot of people are unkind to animals, especially in the name of commerce, the cruelty is condoned and, once large sums of money are at stake, will be defended to the last by otherwise intelligent people."–Ruth Harrison, animal welfare advocate and author of Animal Machines (1920-2000)

FOOD FOR THOUGHT

But I thought eating meat was healthy? Of course you did. Big Ag, the Cattlemen's Association, the American Pork Producers, Poultry Producers, the American Dairy Council, etc. spend huge sums to make you think that eating animal meat is good for you. The Center for Responsive Politics reports that in 2013 agribusiness spent $150 million lobbying Congress.[3] Representatives from these lobbying PACs heavily influence government. They are on the FDA, USDA, supposedly policing the very businesses they profit from. Often, agri-business members sit on governing boards. Yes, it is an obvious conflict of interest. As they say, 'money talks'. When you see an ad encouraging you to drink milk, eat a $1 Hamburger, or add bacon there's ONE reason why- the food industry wants to make money on their product. If you buy it, they will. They don't care for your health; they are an industry. Like all commerce, it all comes down to the bottom line. The more you eat, the more animal products consumed and sold, the more money they make. The more animals they can cram into a tiny space, the faster they can grow and get to slaughter, the more profit is made. Agribusiness ignores your well-being. Agribusiness will graze cattle on government land and even get our government agencies to kill off whatever was living there, such as bison, wild horses or wolves. Due to political influence, our government subsidizes the cost of feed corn and other crops fed to animals rendering greater profits. According to the Washington Post, the farm bill passed in July 2013 subsidizes billions to farmers. It's a business.[4] A very profitable business. Most food is advertised for the sole purpose of making money- like any other business. If you see a food being advertised on network television keep in mind that the intent is to get you to buy it so the company makes money.

FOOD SAFETY

In 1993 America had the first widely publicized e. coli deaths and subsequent ground beef recalls due to e. coli contamination. Escherichia coli/E. Coli is found in feces. Feces are in or on most any animal meat product. Cooking a burger past medium rare, or cooking a chicken beyond pink doesn't destroy the e. coli (or the feces) - it just makes the e. coli bacteria count below levels lethal to humans. Some fecal matter and E.coli are still on and in the meat, but they are warmed or somewhat cooked.

The latest Mad Cow (Bovine spongiform encephalopathy/BSE) outbreak was spread by feeding cows other ground up infected cows. Cows and sheep which were known to be diseased and thus unfit for human consumption were ground up and fed to non-diseased cows. These cows were subsequently consumed by people. Cows which are natural herbivores are also fed other animal waste, such as dead dogs and cats, poultry, and cattle blood. Since the last outbreak, the USDA does not allow dead cows to be fed to live cows. Instead, cattle waste is fed to chickens, and chicken waste is fed to cattle.

Chicken litter, which is a mixture of dead chickens mixed with feathers and chicken manure is regularly fed to cows.[5]

Chickens are sometimes infected with bird flu, which is easily transmitted in overcrowded conditions. Chicken also often contains salmonella. The chicken has e. coli from fecal matter, which is why it is standard industry practice to dip the parts into ammonia or bleach solution before packaging. Consumer Reports 2014 study of more than 300 raw chicken breasts found that 10.8% had salmonella, while 65.2% tested positive for E. coli. Overall, about 97% of the breasts tested contained harmful bacteria, according to that study.[6]

In 2014 Congress passed a law privatizing poultry inspection. Most USDA inspectors will be replaced by company employees and processing speeds will increase. This means more industry self-policing and fewer government inspectors, in an industry which just was found to have harmful bacteria levels in nearly ALL the meat samples.[7]

A Consumer Reports study found 69% of pork chops and ground pork sampled from around the U.S. tested positive for Yersinia enterocolitica. The bacteria can cause fever, abdominal pain and diarrhea, according to the Centers for Disease Control and Prevention.[8]

Farmed fish are primarily fed fecal matter (chicken and pig feces). Wild caught fish are subject to ocean pollution and are affected by nuclear Fukushima's radiation leak. A recent study from Oregon State University has shown that radiation in albacore tuna caught off the Oregon coast tripled after the 2011 Fukushima nuclear meltdown in Japan.[9]

In 2014 the consumption of animal meat was found to contribute to the spread of the Ebola virus. 'Bush meat' from carrier animals was transmitted to people. 'Bush meat' is flesh from monkeys and bats.[10]

There have been massive and multiple recalls of animal products in 2014 alone. Reasons for recalls ranged from various contaminations to lack of inspections. Some of these recall quantities have numbered in the thousands of tons of animal meat.[11]

Animals are fed animal waste, antibiotics and hormones. After slaughter the flesh contains feces, antibiotics and hormones. Garbage in, garbage out. No wonder that impartial studies and inspections have found massive quantities of unsafe animal products in our food supply.

"Nothing will benefit human health and increase the chances for survival of life on earth as much as the evolution to a vegetarian diet."–Albert Einstein, theoretical physicist and philosopher of science. (1879-1955)

HEART HEALTH

Heart attacks are the number one killer of firefighters.[12] In fact, heart disease is the number one cause of death for all Americans. Lifestyle, notably diet, is the number one cause of heart disease. Consuming animal fats and animal products are the greatest contributor to heart disease. Diet is crucial to your health or lack thereof. Heart disease is preventable and correctable.[13]

If the number one threat to your life is a heart attack (and it is) stop eating animals. What?! Give up meat? But animals taste so delicious...Yes, I know it's scary. I have not always been on a plant-based diet. It's not the flavor of meat that I found a problem with, it is everything else. Don't let your taste buds dictate your health. They will adjust. Nutrition should be your dietary guide. After all, food is fuel for your body. The food you choose can build health, or it can contribute to disease conditions.

The China Study, by T. Colin Campbell, PhD and Dr. Thomas M. Campbell II examines the relationship between the consumption of animal products and chronic illnesses such as coronary heart disease, diabetes, and cancer. The authors conclude that people who eat a whole-food, vegan plant-based diet can prevent, reduce and reverse the development of numerous diseases.[14]

Staying heart healthy is a great way to avoid being that next heart attack on a call. You don't want to risk the lives of your brothers and sisters due to a Mayday. I'm sure you'd rather remain an asset than a detriment to your crew, your department, and your family. We don't want to read about your demise on the Secret List.[15] There are already far too many heart attacks every single year, 2014 included. Heart disease is reversible with lifestyle changes. A diet free from animal fats along with regular exercise will keep your blood flowing freely.

"And God said, 'Behold, I have given you every herb bearing seed, which is on the face of all the earth, and every tree, in which is the fruit of a tree yielding seed; to you it shall be for meat.'" –The Bible, Genesis 1:29

CANCER

The number two killer of all Americans- half of us will get cancer of some type.[16] There are runs 'for the cure', pink ribbons 'for the cure', many numerous foundations and research 'for the cure'. One answer is found on our plate. In addition to using proper PPE and washing carcinogens from gear, we can reduce the carcinogens that we eat. The American Institute for Cancer Research proclaims, 'our bottom-line message is the same: Diets that revolve around whole plant foods – vegetables, whole grains, fruits and beans – cut the risk of many cancers, and other diseases as well.'[17] Researcher Dr. Dean Ornish and his team showed that men eating plant based diet for a year had 8 times the amount of cancer fighting compounds in their bloodstream.[18]

A 2012 study, 'Annals of Nutrition and Metabolism' study found that vegetarians have lower cancer rates than the general population. Research shows that vegetarians are about fifty percent less likely to develop cancer than those who eat meat.[19] The University of Southern California found in 2014 that a diet high in animal proteins may be as bad as smoking in terms of increasing cancer risk.[20] Don't want cancer, diabetes and heart disease? Then eat like you mean it.

HYDRAULICS

Erectile dysfunction is often one of the earliest symptoms of circulatory problems.[21] The penis is an organ whose performance is based on blood flow. A problem that you see the urologist for is one you probably should be seeing a cardiologist for. Or, did you think that your body had a naturally occurring blue pill deficiency? Blood flow becomes impeded at the penis and other extremities when vessels are clogged with animal fats and arterial buildup. It's easier to notice in the penis, well, first of all, because you're looking, and secondly, because the vein system is smaller and finer than the larger heart arteries and veins. Quit putting animal products in your mouth and you'll happily see that things start looking up again...without the need for erectile dysfunction drugs. There will be no need to wait- but instead a welcome return to spontaneity.

Male firefighters are usually popular with the ladies. Animal lovers also get points with the ladies. Vegetarians, ditto. Imagine the combination.

Compassion is always attractive, and so is vibrant health.

PREVENTION

You know how fires aren't what they used to be? These days they are much more synthetic and plastic and dangerous. We rely on Prevention to insist on sprinklers and plans and standpipes because we've learned and we're smarter now. Prevention is the key to limiting damage before it even occurs. Let Prevention be your guide. Remember how the best fire is the one that never happens? Take a tip from the Prevention Division. Preventing heart disease to begin with is easier and cheaper than open heart surgery, bypasses, or treatment with hazardous drugs.

Stents and drugs are meant to be a temporary solution. If drugs really were the key to good health, then wouldn't our healthiest patients be the ones on the most medications? If drugs truly cured their conditions, then people who take multiple medications would look and truly be healthy. Instead they make up our best EMS customers- frequent fliers with long lists of medications. Learn from your own observations in the field. You can improve your overall foundation, and get your blood flowing properly. Your circulation will be improved when your blood is not all gummed up with animal fat and cholesterol. If you don't put it into your mouth, it can't get onto your arterial walls.

Plant based diet a little too extreme for you? 'What do you call 500,000 people each year having their chest opened up on an operating table, and having a vein from their leg sewn onto their heart?' responds Dr. Caldwell Esselstyn, in the documentary 'Forks Over Knives'.[22]

It is alarming that heart attacks continue to be the number one killer of firefighters. It is sad that half of our American population will die of heart disease. Half of all Americans will get cancer. So far, most of us have not utilized the tools available to prevent or postpone our own demise.

"...believe that compassion, in which all ethics must take root, can only attain its full breadth and depth if it embraces all living creatures and does not limit itself to mankind."—Albert Schweitzer, theologian, philosopher, physician, and medical missionary (1875-1965)

EVEN HEROES HAVE COGNITIVE DISSONANCE

Firefighters, EMTs, paramedics and police officers are some of the kindest people I know. I have heard stories of their kindness dating back to childhood. With hearts so big they wanted to help others and serve mankind by becoming First Responders. I've heard many a story of baby birds rescued from fallen nests, homeless animals fed, and strays adopted. Most of our pets are some kind of rescue or adoption. I've been called to rescue baby squirrels, ducks, possums, dogs and cats. Our fire department has rescued baby ducks, dogs, cats, birds. Many fire departments have rescued dogs and cats from confined spaces, fires and other hazardous situations. Some departments do large animal rescue. So why are we helping some animals and eating others? Saving baby ducklings then dining on chicken wings? This perplexing behavior is because of cognitive dissonance.

Cognitive dissonance is when we hold two incompatible thoughts at the same time. An example of this would be a person that knows smoking is bad for health, but continues to smoke cigarettes. "When dissonance is present, in addition to trying to reduce it, the person will actively avoid situations and information which would likely increase the dissonance," according to psychologist Leon Festinger, author of A Theory of Cognitive Dissonance.[23] We believe we are kind, caring people. We say we love animals. We purchase and consume animal products which are a result of inhumane factory farming and slaughter. We then purposely avoid information and situations that would make us examine that contradiction, to remain more comfortable psychologically. We have internal dialogue that dismisses facts and uncomfortable feelings. Examples of the internal dialogue of the smoker could be- 'well, I won't get cancer' or 'if I quit smoking I might get fat' or 'hey, you have to die of something'.

The internal dialogue of a meat eater may be 'well, I won't get cancer' or 'I love meat' or 'hey, you have to die of something' or even 'eh, I don't believe all these medical studies'. This type of rationalization and denial helps balance the dissonant thoughts. We like to believe that we are consistent with our beliefs and behavior. But we are not.

SAVING LIVES

Why is a barn fire one of the most horrific things ever- but a barbeque is great? Both really involve the horrendous suffering and burnt flesh of animals. Why save Mr. Smith's parakeet, but eat Mr. Purdue's chicken? The oath we've all taken. We answer the question, 'why do you want to be a firefighter?' with 'I want to save lives and preserve property'. Animals are living beings, they think and feel. They have family, friends and intelligence. A pig is smarter than a dog. They have as much intelligence as a 3-year-old child.[24] Animals raised in factory conditions suffer tremendously during their lives, and horribly during their deaths. 99% of all farmed animals come from factory farms. 'Factory farms' are a far cry from the family farms of the past. They are much closer to a factory and are known as Concentrated Animal Feeding Operations or CAFOs.[25]

Many of us carry ventilation masks on our apparatus for the purpose of saving an animals life. Some fire departments have teams who specialize in large animal rescue. If we are going to save Mr. Smith's parakeet, Mrs. Jones' cat, and little Billy's pot-bellied pig- doesn't it make sense that we spare the chicken, the cow and the pig from suffering industrial factory farm conditions and a gruesome death?

We can save other people's lives by skipping meat. According to the United Nations, 21,000 people die of hunger or hunger related causes each day. This equals one person dying of hunger every four seconds, most of whom are children.[26] Meanwhile, we are feeding corn and other crops to fatten cattle, pork, and chicken. This animal fodder could be saving starving people instead of fattening up our pork chops.

Of course, by skipping animal meat we would save animal lives. Since the 1970s we have killed off half the animal species on earth. Half of animal species in the last 44 years has gone extinct by overfishing and overhunting, habitat degradation and climate change.[27]

Not only are entire species decimated by our appetite. Each year we kill 70 billion land animals for food alone.[28] A person on a plant based diet saves an average of 100 animal lives a year. For more information on land animals, birds, fish and shellfish spared by vegetarians, see: Counting Animals.[29] You can save more lives with a dietary change than you can in your entire career!

"People care about animals. I believe that. They just don't want to know or to pay. A fourth of all chickens have stress fractures. It's wrong. They're packed body to body, and can't escape their waste, and never see the sun. Their nails grow around the bars of their cages. It's wrong. They feel their slaughters. It's wrong, and people know it's wrong. They don't have to be convinced. They just have to act differently. I'm not better than anyone, and I'm not trying to convince people to live by my standards of what's right. I'm trying to convince them to live by their own."– *Jonathan Safran Foer, author of Everything Is Illuminated; Eating Animals; and Extremely Loud and Incredibly Close (1977-)*

CHICKEN?

The life of a male chicken ends abruptly upon discovery that he is a male. Baby chicks are sorted by employees called 'sexers' who determine their gender of female and male. Male chicks then go into a grinder, alive, or put in a garbage bag with all their brethren to suffocate. Sometimes they are killed by electrocution. Since male chickens cannot lay eggs, they cannot be 'layers'. Female chickens have been determined to be more plump and juicy than males, so the male chick is calculated to be a poor investment. Upon further examination of the life of his sister, immediate death may be the better way out. Overcrowding is part of the profit margin lifestyle. A chicken will peck other chickens when they are squashed, crowded, stressed and aggravated by other chickens, with no room to go to. Rather than give them decent space, their beaks are cut. The young layer hen goes into what's called a 'battery' cage. A battery cage is about the size of your Kindle. She just exists in there, can't move, and cannot open her wings. The caged chickens are kept in the dark, with little air circulation. Saving electricity adds to the profit margin. Cages are stacked on top of each other. Picture a hangar sized warehouse with rows upon rows of cages, that's the current chicken factory farm.

Conditions are such to make the chickens sicken and die, which they do, in great numbers. And rather than improve living conditions so they can survive, agribusiness finds it cheaper to give them drugs. In fact, 70% of antibiotics used in the world are for animal agriculture. The industry tries to keep most of the creatures alive long enough to reach the slaughterhouse. When the birds are being transported to slaughter, they go without food or water. They suffer temperature extremes from blazing summer heat to freezing winter blizzards. Most slaughterhouses/processing plants are somewhat isolated and chickens will travel for days. Many will be DOA, many will have suffered injuries such as broken legs and wings. The slaughter process is also designed to make a profit including mechanized processes, low staffing levels of unskilled labor. Inspectors are few and limited. Many chickens go through the process alive. The chickens move about while on the processing line. They often miss the line throat slitter, and are scalded alive. According to the National Chicken Council, about 180 million chickens are improperly slaughtered each year. All poultry is exempt from the minimal protections offered by The Humane Methods of Slaughter Act.[30] As consumers we continue to support these industry practices with our purchasing dollars. We vote with our wallets.

"Let food be thy medicine."–Hippocrates, Greek physician and father of western medicine (460-370 BC)

THE ROOKIE'S IN CHARGE?

Putting your taste buds in charge of what fuels your body is like putting the rookie in charge of the fire engine. Yes, s/he thinks he knows a lot, but really, putting an overconfident kid in charge of a half-million-dollar fire engine would be considered poor judgment by most. So is putting your taste buds in charge of what vitamins, minerals and other nutrients your body needs. The good news is that your taste buds- like your rookie- are trainable. You have to teach them what is truly important. They will adapt. Food is fuel, and you can eat for health or disease. Your taste buds will only take about 2 weeks to adapt. Simple and fresh foods will become enjoyable to you. Fruits and vegetables are great for your overall health. Eating animal meat will become as distasteful as the idea of eating a grilled kitten sandwich. You will enjoy the bounty of a plant based diet, and you will enjoy your improved health. There are many products and lots of information to help you transition during this brief period, such as Mercy for Animals' free starter kit.[31]

You know what a huge mistake it would be to put gasoline into the hydraulic fluid tank of your extrication equipment, right? It would be hours of costly labor, and expensive parts to repair the lines and motor. (Not to mention some yelling). Treat your body like a priceless piece of equipment that cannot be replaced. Don't put animal products into it, then you won't have to repair the resulting damage.

PRESERVING PROPERTY

A third of the earth is used for livestock, according to the United Nation's Food and Agriculture Organization. One-third of our planet's prime land is dedicated to producing animal meat. The 70 Billion land animals that are killed each year for food need to be housed, fed, transported to slaughter, slaughtered, butchered, packaged and transported to consumers. 99% of these animals are from a Concentrated Animal Feeding Operation (CAFO), an industrial-sized livestock operation. Although crowded in a CAFO, millions of acres are required due to the sheer quantity of animals required for our current appetite.[32]

The Amazon Rainforest, considered the 'lungs of the earth' has been cleared to make grazing land for cattle. The Amazon is the biggest source of oxygen for the planet. 91% of the clearing is due to animal agriculture. It is being cleared at the rate of 1-2 acres per second.[33]

The amount of water used for animal agriculture is tremendous. The meat and dairy industries use almost one third of all fresh water in the world. Many look to animal agriculture as causing continuing droughts. Each pound of beef requires about 2,500 gallons of water to produce. If the cost of water weren't subsidized by taxpayers, a pound of hamburger would cost over $35 a pound in water usage alone. To compare- a pound of apples requires 83 gallons of water to produce and a pound of potatoes requires 20 gallons of water to produce. People are encouraged to conserve water during drought by limiting personal usage, but a person would save more water just by replacing one pound of beef with plant foods than by not showering for two months.[34]

Animal agriculture is a major cause of groundwater pollution. Animals produce about 130 times more excrement than the entire human population every year. Unlike human waste, animal waste is not processed as sewage. These huge cesspools of waste pollute the land, often seeping through the soil and contaminating water. The amount of urine and feces from even the tiniest CAFO equals the urine and feces produced from a small city. In United States animal excrement from CAFOs has contaminated groundwater in 17 states and polluted 35,000 miles of rivers in 22 states.[35]

So, a third of the earth, a third of the world's grain, a third of the world's water supply devoted to animal agriculture. The cost of these resources is subsidized by taxpayers. In their wake, the factory farms leave massive leaky lagoons of untreated animal waste. If a third of your house was being wrecked, with raw sewage left in exchange, you would be doing something about it, pronto! A third of our land and water is being wrecked, and our dietary choices can massively reduce the destruction.

"If slaughterhouses had glass walls, everyone would be vegetarian." Sir Paul McCartney, animal rights activist, singer/songwriter for The Beatles (1942-)

GOOD COMPANY

Hopefully you take pride in your company, your crew, your house. You may catch some flak for your new way of eating. Rest assured you are in good company. Not just the Roman Gladiators were vegetarian. Once you go plant-based, you can join some of the world leaders, geniuses, celebrities, and world class champion athletes such as these: Environmental advocate (former) Vice President Al Gore; scientist Albert Einstein; theologian/philosopher and physician Albert Schweitzer; writer Alice Walker; actress/author Alicia Silverstone; NASCAR driver Andy Lally; actor and animal advocate Anthony Hopkins; NBA athlete Anthony Peeler; writer/speaker Anthony Robbins; Greek philosopher Aristotle; musician BB King; pediatrician and author Dr. Benjamin Spock; actress Betty White; (former) President Bill Clinton; NBA All-Star Bill Walton; tennis legend Billie Jean King; singer Beyoncé; TV host and animal advocate Bob Barker; actor Brad Pitt; athlete Brendan Brazier; Olympic champion and United Nations Goodwill Ambassador Carl Lewis; country singer Carrie Underwood; actress Carrie Anne Moss; radio/TV host Casey Kasem; United Farm Workers labor leader Cesar Chavez; Rolling Stones drummer Charlie Watts; tennis legend Chris Evert; Coldplay lead singer/musician Chris Martin; singer Chrissie Hynde; actor Christian Bale; supermodel Christie Brinkley; supermodel Claudia Schiffer; activist Martin Luther King Jr.'s widow Coretta Scott King; actress and environmental activist Daryl Hannah; Ironman world champion Dave Scott; NFL player David Carter; author Dr. Deepak Chopra; musician Dizzie Gillespie; actor and rights activist Ed Asner; singer/Pearl Jam songwriter Eddie Vedder; actor Edward Furlong; TV host Ellen Degeneres; Greek philosopher Epicurus; Olympic athlete Fiona Oakes; writer Franz Kafka; Hindu Spiritual leader Gandhi; writer George Bernard Shaw; NHL player George Laraque; writer Harriet Beecher Stowe; former cattle rancher turned author/activist Howard Lyman; actor Ian McKellan; director James Cameron; actor and animal rights activist James Cromwell; comedian Jamie Kennedy;

actress Jamie Lee Curtis; primatologist/educator and animal rights advocate Jane Goodall; actor/singer Jared Leto; writer JD Salinger; guitarist Jeff Beck; mystic/saint Rabbi Jesus Christ; musician Joan Jett; actor Joaquin Phoenix; NFL athlete Joe Namath; The Beatles musician John Lennon; physician/author Dr. John McDougall; author and activist John Robbins; NBA champion John Salley; author Jonathan Safran Foer; actor Keenen Ivory Wayans; singer Kelly Clarkson; pro surfer Ken Bradshaw; (former) President of Zambia Dr. Kenneth Kaunda; professional wrestler Killer Kowalski; actress Kim Basinger; musician/Nirvana bassist Krist Novoselic; actor Larry Hagman; Russian writer/philosopher Leo Tolstoy; Italian painter/inventor Leonardo Da Vinci; actress Linda Carter; actress Lindsay Wagner; author Louisa May Alcott; UFC ultimate fighter Luke Cummo; actress/author Marilu Henner; comedian Marty Feldman; actress Mary Tyler Moore; singer Michael Jackson; athlete, author/actor Mike Tyson; author/musician Moby; singer Morrissey; TV host/educator Mr. (Fred) Rogers; Prime Minister of India Narendra Modi; actress Natalie Portman; physicist/inventor Nikola Tesla; director Oliver Stone; actress Pamela Anderson; NBA athlete Pau

Gasol; The Beatles musician Sir Paul McCartney; singer/songwriter Peter Gabriel; comedian Peter Sellers; musician/Grateful Dead bass player Phil Lesh; singer Pink; Greek philosopher Plato; musician Prince; Greek mathematician (Pythagorean Theorem) Pythagoras of Samos; NBA athlete Raja Bell; writer Ralph Waldo Emerson; NFL athlete Ricky Williams; The Beatles musician Ringo Starr; musician/film director Rob Zombie; actor/film producer Robert Redford; NBA Hall-of-Famer Robert Parish; The Cure musician Robert Smith; civil rights activist Rosa Parks; music producer and Def Records co-founder Russell Simmons; friar and official Patron of Ecology Saint/San Francesco d'Assisi; actor Samuel L. Jackson; singer/songwriter Seal; Olympian athlete, actress/writer Seba Johnson; singer Shania Twain; physicist Sir Isaac Newton; Greek philosopher Socrates; women's suffrage pioneer Susan B. Anthony; music band The Roots; inventor Thomas Edison; Motley Crue musician Tommy Lee; Major League Baseball coach and animal advocate Tony La Russa; Grand Slam tennis champion Venus Williams; French writer/philosopher Voltaire; actor and environmental activist Woody Harrelson.

Most of this list and many more can be found here: https://www.happycow.net/vegtopics/famous.[36] Join champion athletes, world leaders and innovators-the healthy, smart and soulful who have made the world a better place not just with their works, but also with their forks.

"Humanity's true moral test, its fundamental test…consists of its attitude towards those who are at its mercy: animals."— Milan Kundera, author of The Unbearable Lightness of Being (1929-)

HEROES ARE ROLE MODELS

A firefighter is a role model in the community- a step above, hopefully a good example. Candidates are weeded out with rigorous physical examinations and testing, questionnaires, background checks and interviews. There is no person or profession more respected and trusted than a firefighter, according to American polls. Keys to the city, entrance to all homes. We are 'the good guys'. The public is highly interested in us –let us be a good example in the way we eat, the way we show compassion, the way we take responsibility for our own health. The public watches our every move, they wear our t-shirts and watch movies and television shows about us. They watch us in the grocery store. Little kids want to be us when they grow up. The majority of our public does not live an active lifestyle. Our community may see us chowing down on ribs and burgers and think it's a good idea, because we are doing it. Since we have firefighter inspired restaurants, condiments, even cooking shows, they know we can eat- but can we eat right? Let us show them the way by a positive healthy example. Be a good leader in the community by setting the example in your actions. Cook veggies when it's your turn to cook at the station, share your knowledge. Often, people aren't quite sure what to eat when skipping the meat. Show your brothers and sisters that you truly care about their health by feeding them healthy fare. Cook them veggie burgers, salad, pasta primavera, steamed, roasted, grilled and baked vegetables. There are many animal meat substitutes. Be ahead of the curve. When you have events with the public, continue to be positive role models. Provide healthy refreshments at open houses or health expos. Put that phrase of 'saving lives and protecting property' into action on a daily dietary basis. Remember the Prevention model when it comes to diet and health. People really do look to us for us as role models in every way. When they look at you, your crew, and your department- do they see people who rescue some animals but eat others? Or do they see trim, fit people who are respecting their own health? Do they see people who are conserving resources by consuming a plant based diet?

"There is a principle which is a bar against all information, which is proof against all argument, and which cannot fail to keep a man in everlasting ignorance. This principle is contempt prior to examination." – William Paley, philosopher (1743-1805)

ADAPT AND OVERCOME!

There was a time when all people believed the earth was flat. Doctors used to smoke cigarettes. Riding tailboard was standard. Eating animal products was thought to be healthy, not carcinogenic. 'Eating smoke' was common. As we gain information, we change and improve. We improve our tactics, and adopt new ones. You are the most valuable tool on the truck, and we need you. We need you educated, fit and healthy. If you are the 'heart attack waiting to happen' you are jeopardizing your crew. If you go down, you know we will go after you to get you, or die trying. You've got nothing to lose by trying a plant based diet. You can test this dietary approach on yourself. Get a full physical including bloodwork. Then eat a plant-based diet for one month. Get another checkup and compare your results. If you don't look and feel better, with better hydraulics, and bloodwork-you can always go back to eating animals. My best friend, another firefighter, changed to a plant-based diet after a heart scare, which included a hypovolemic incident. Now, he's dropped weight, cut one blood pressure medication, and eliminated another medication.

Be first in. You can do this, too! You now have the facts about the importance of food and your health. You know the consequences of your dietary decisions for your crew, your family and your community. Make the world a better place. Join the winners who eat like heroes, with help for your 30-day transition.[37] Afraid to go all in? You can start with Meatless Mondays.[38] Also, you can check out the website eatlikeahero.com for more inspiration and information. Please share your review of this book on Amazon. Share your success stories with your friends and fire family on Facebook and Twitter. Enjoy in good health, and always stay safe.

ABOUT THE AUTHOR

As a child Andrea Laurel lived on a dairy farm and was involved with agriculture clubs such as 4-H and Future Farmers of America. Her first jobs were in Foodservice. She stayed in the business and received her Bachelor of Science degree in Hospitality in 1991. She has worked in the Foodservice profession for over 30 years, in restaurants, catering, clubs and hotels. Always interested in food and marketing, she has learned much about food over the past three decades, not just from professors, but in real world practices. In 2006 she became a certified combat active firefighter with the Plantation Fire Department and later became a certified Emergency Medical Technician-Basic. Her knowledge of food and firefighters led her to write this rationale to inspire her fellow firefighters to adopt a plant based diet.

SOURCES:

[1] Mills, Milton R., M.D. "The Comparative Anatomy of Eating." *Vegsource.com*. VegSource Interactive, November 21, 2009. Educational website.

http://www.vegsource.com/news/2009/11/the-comparative-anatomy-of-eating.html

[2] "The Protein Myth." *Physician's Committee for Responsible Medicine*. Pcrm.org, December 2014. Informational website.

http://pcrm.org/health/diets/vsk/vegetarian-starter-kit-protein

[3] "Annual Lobbying on Agribusiness." Center for Responsive Politics, October 27, 2014. Non-profit organization website.

https://www.opensecrets.org/lobby/indus.php?id=A

[4] Editorial Board. "In Congress's Farm Bill the Rich Get Richer." The Washington Post, February 4, 2014. News website.

http://www.washingtonpost.com/opinions/in-congresss-farm-bill-the-rich-get-richer/2014/02/04/331443a8-8dd7-11e3-833c-33098f9e5267_story.html

[5] Mercola, Joseph O., DO/Dr. "Is the Meat You Are Eating Being Fed Animal Feces?" Mercola.com, June 20, 2012. Informational website.

> http://articles.mercola.com/sites/articles/archive/2012/06/30/chicken-litter-causes-mad-cow-disease.aspx

[6] ConsumerReports.org. "The High Cost Of Cheap Chicken." *Consumer Reports Magazine*, January 2014. Consumer education website.

> http://www.consumerreports.org/cro/magazine/2014/02/the-high-cost-of-cheap-chicken/index.htm

[7] "Consumer and Worker Rights Groups File Amicus in Opposition of New Poultry Inspection System." *Food Integrity Campaign*, October 3, 2014. Whistleblower organization website.

> http://www.foodwhistleblower.org/consumer-and-worker-rights-groups-file-amicus-in-opposition-of-new-poultry-inspection-system

[8] Newcomb, Alyssa. "Study Finds Most Pork Contaminated With Yersinia Bacteria." ABC.com, November 2012. News website.

> http://abcnews.go.com/blogs/health/2012/11/27/study-finds-most-pork-contaminated-with-yersinia-bacteria

52

9 ENENews. "USA Today: Radiation tripled in some albacore tuna off West Coast after Fukushima — Bioaccumulating in bones, not only flesh." *News Network*, April 29, 2014. News website.

>http://enenews.com/usa-today-radiation-tripled-in-some-albacore-tuna-off-west-coast-after-fukushima-bioaccumulation-occuring-in-bones-not-only-flesh-additional-exposures-to-plume-could-further-increase-radiati

10 National Center for Emerging and Zoonotic Infectious Diseases, "Facts about Bushmeat and Ebola." *Centers for Disease Control Fact Sheet*, September 2014. Government Health and Safety Information website.

>http://www.cdc.gov/vhf/ebola/pdf/bushmeat-and-ebola.pdf

11 Department of Agriculture/USDA, "Current Recalls and Alerts." *Food Safety and Inspection Service Public Health Alerts*, updated June 30, 2016. Government food safety website.

>http://www.fsis.usda.gov/wps/portal/fsis/topics/recalls-and-public-health-alerts/current-recalls-and-alerts

12 Federal Emergency Management Agency. "Firefighter Fatalities Statistics and Reports." *U. S. Fire Administration/USFA*, updated October 9, 2014. Government safety administration website.

>https://www.usfa.fema.gov/data/statistics

[13] "Lifestyle Changes for Heart Attack Prevention." *American Heart Association*, updated October 20, 2012. Non-profit health information website.

http://www.heart.org/HEARTORG/Conditions/HeartAttack/PreventionTreatmentofHeartAttack/Lifestyle-Changes_UCM_303934_Article.jsp

[14] Parker-Pope, Tara. "Nutrition Advice From the China Study." *The New York Times*, Published January 7, 2011. News website blog.

http://well.blogs.nytimes.com/2011/01/07/nutrition-advice-from-the-china-study/?_r=0

[15] Goldfeder, Billy, Chief. "The Secret List." *FirefighterCloseCalls.com*, established 1998.

http://firefighterclosecalls.com/category/secret-list

(included with permission of Chief Billy Goldfeder).

[16] Centers for Disease Control and Prevention. "Leading Causes of Death (final 2014 data)." *National Center for Health Statistics FastStats,* updated April 27 2016. Government health website.

http://www.cdc.gov/nchs/fastats/leading-causes-of-death.htm

[17] American Institute for Cancer Research. "Diet - What We Eat." *Reduce Your Cancer Risk,* published 2016. Research news website.

http://www.aicr.org/reduce-your-cancer-risk/diet

[18] Greger, Michael, M.D. "Cancer-Proofing Your Body." *NutritionFacts.org,* Dr. Greger's Medical Nutrition Blog, published January 2013. Nutrition research website.

http://nutritionfacts.org/2013/01/31/cancer-proofing-your-body

[19] Paul, Maya W., Smith, Melinda, M.A., and Robinson, Lawrence. "Cancer Prevention Diet – Lower Your Risk with Cancer-Fighting Foods." *Helpguide.org,* updated February 2016. Non-profit wellness website.

http://www.helpguide.org/articles/diet-weight-loss/anti-cancer-diet.htm

[20] University of Southern California. "Meat and cheese may be as bad for you as smoking." *ScienceDaily.com*, March 4, 2014. Research news website.

http://www.sciencedaily.com/releases/2014/03/140304125639.htm

[21] Patrick J. Skerrett. "Erectile Dysfunction Often a Warning Sign of Heart Disease." *Harvard Medical Schools Harvard Health Blog*, October 24, 2011. Medical news website blog.

http://www.health.harvard.edu/blog/erectile-dysfunction-often-a-warning-sign-of-heart-disease-201110243648

[22] Frazier, Matt. "Forks Over Knives." *No Meat Athlete Film Review Blog*, May 2011. Fitness website blog.

http://www.nomeatathlete.com/forks-over-knives-review/#sthash.NcDfrmq9.dpuf

[23] McLeod, Saul. "Cognitive Dissonance." *Simply Psychology*, updated 2014. Psychology information website.

http://www.simplypsychology.org/cognitive-dissonance.html

[24] Wright, Andy. "Pigheaded: How Smart are Swine?" *Modern Farmer Media*, March 10 2014. Farming information website.

http://modernfarmer.com/2014/03/pigheaded-smart-swine

[25] "Factory Farming." *Farm Forward*, 2016.Online advocacy newsletter.

http://www.farmforward.com/farming-forward/factory-farming

[26] Kruth, Caressa. "Should 21,000 Deaths from Global Poverty Matter to the U.S.? *The Borgen Project, The Blog*, September 2013. Non-profit organization website.

http://borgenproject.org/21000-deaths-global-poverty-matter-u-s

[27] Ingraham, Christopher. "We've Killed Off Half the Worlds Animals Since 1970." *Washington Post Wonkblog*, September 30, 2014. News website.

http://www.washingtonpost.com/blogs/wonkblog/wp/2014/09/30/weve-killed-off-half-the-worlds-animals-since-1970

28 "HSI Calls on Global Leaders to Adopt Meatless Mondays." *Humane Society International*, September 12, 2012. Animal welfare website.

http://www.hsi.org/news/press_releases/2012/09/meatless _mondays_hungerforaction_conference_091212.html

29 Harish,"How Many Animals Does a Vegetarian Save?" *Counting Animals,* updated February 22, 2012. Animal advocacy website.

http://www.countinganimals.com/how-many-animals-does-a-vegetarian-save

30 Foer, Jonathan Safran *Eating Animals*. New York, NY: Little, Brown and Company, 2010. Print.

31 "Order a Free Vegetarian Starter Guide." *Mercy for Animals*, 2016. Non-profit advocacy and informational website.

http://www.chooseveg.com/free-veg-guide

32 Oppenlander, Richard A. *Food Choice and Sustainability: Why Buying Local, Eating Less Meat, and Taking Baby Steps Won't Work*. Minneapolis, MN: Langdon Street, 2013. Print.

33 *Cowspiracy: The Sustainability Secret*, 2014, Film.

34 Catanese, Christina. "Virtual Water, Real Impacts." *Greenversations: Official Blog of the U.S. Environmental Protection Agency*. 2012. Government agency website.

http://blog.epa.gov/healthywaters/2012/03/virtual-water-real-impacts-world-water-day-2012

35 "Factory Farm Pollution." *Food Empowerment Project*, 2014. Non-profit food justice organization website.

http://www.foodispower.org/pollution-water-air-chemicals

36 "Veg Topics: Famous Vegans and Vegetarians." *Happy Cow,The Healthy Eating Guide*, updated 2016.

https://www.happycow.net/vegtopics/famous

37 "Order a Free Vegetarian Starter Guide." *Mercy for Animals*, 2014. Non-profit advocacy and informational website.

http://www.chooseveg.com/free-veg-guide

38 "Meatless Monday Recipes." *Meatless Monday*, updated 2016. Nutritional campaign website.

http://www.meatlessmonday.com/favorite-recipes

48582347N00039

Made in the USA
Columbia, SC
12 January 2019